The Best Anti Aging Diet. Ever!

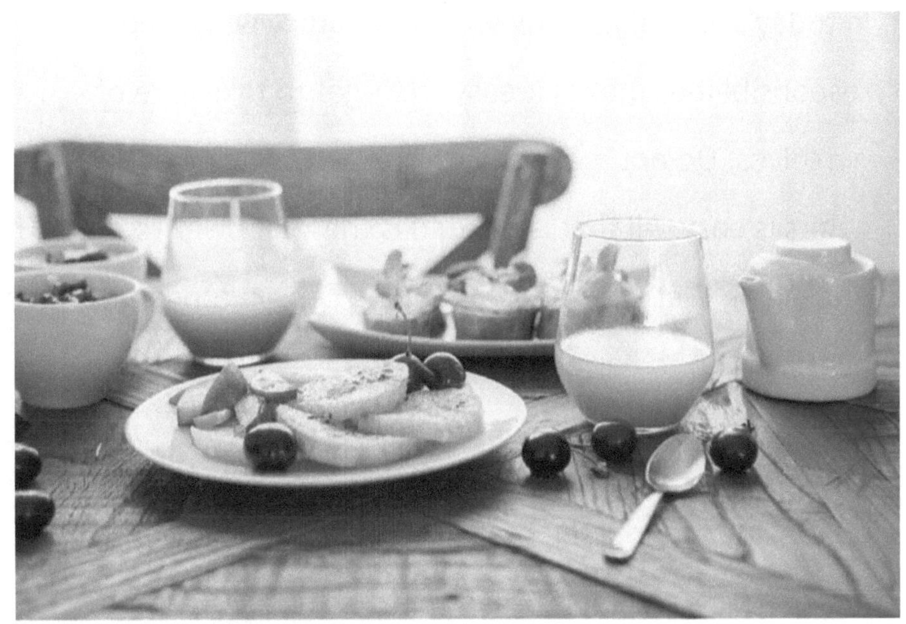

The Importance of Diet for Healthy Aging

Let's face it; when you eat right, your body has energy and nutrients to maintain your health. In addition to eating correctly, when you maintain a healthy weight, you decrease your risk of type 2 diabetes and other serious metabolic disorders like heart disease, aches, and pains of the joints, and ailments that result from obesity. You know that a healthy diet is a key to enjoying good health and longer life.

Here is the anti-aging diet in a nutshell

In today's world, juggling work and family with other responsibilities makes it easy to forget to take care of ourselves. Do not make that mistake. Changing eating habits is easy. All that is needed is the willpower to do it. The Anti-Aging Diet is deleting or adding certain foods that have been proven to harm the body.

You do not have to follow any rules that some dude makes up. Decide for yourself how fast or slow to change your eating habits. When I turned to a plant-based diet, the process was simple. I use the term Plant-Based Diet. It is more refined and says it all.

A plant-based diet means what you think it means. I cut out meat whenever I have a choice.

Which I always have, and it is getting bigger every day. I dial back on dairy products and use cashew-based milk in my coffee or tea.

For me, going veggie/plant based, was really easy. I simply stopped ordering meat at restaurants. No chicken or fish either. My daughter, my wife, and I are all veggie heads to varying degrees, and they have been forever, but I was the obstinate one. Whenever there is an option, I choose not to have meat-based products in whatever it was I ate.

I stopped eating processed foods. I still have the occasional chip or sweets. They are not meat based. As an example, when we get hungry, we have a tendency to grab whatever is closest and takes the shortest amount of time to consume. By planning your eating ahead of time, you can make sure to have an assortment of great snacks on hand. Really, its not hard to make little changes in your diet that will greatly affect your health.

Choose oatmeal for breakfast instead of bacon or sausage. You can sprinkle berries on it or add a moderate amount of brown sugar. I still eat the occasional egg, but for ice cream, we eat gluten free and dairy free. They are delicious. You are just substituting. That's all. In place of ordering a hamburger when you go out, pick the one made of plants. They are surprisingly good.

Because we are so swamped and rushed, we lean towards food that has the least nutritional value just to give our taste buds a quick fix. Store bought stuff. We grab fast food and processed snacks draped in pretty wrappings, and we're done with it.

Then, the years start to add up, and we feel sick, exhausted and worn out. Eventually, and a lot sooner than you think, our bodies have had enough and can't keep up anymore. We begin to feel the toll of all our bad choices. Since technology and the media has programmed us to never wait for anything, we search for a quick fix for to our exhaustion so we can return to our busy schedules.

As a consequence, people turn to "magic pills," and quick diet fixes hoping to make the health problems brought on by years of poor diet disappear. They will take a further toll on our health, and instead of feeling good quickly, things will start to go downhill pretty fast.

The good news is that there is a better, more effective way to be healthy, fit, and stay that way. The key to anti-againg. The only catch is that it requires time, attention and consistency. That's it! Think of it as an investment towards your health, and you'll reap the returns in enjoying vitality and good health as the years go by.

Growing old is inevitable. You can't escape from it. However, by making smarter choices when it comes to what you eat and drink, you can add many years to your life. This book will show you how to apply an anti-aging diet.

While it's true that there are numerous variables as to how we age, it has been scientifically proven that by following a healthy lifestyle that includes a well-balanced diet and regular exercise you can slow down the aging process and ward off lifestyle diseases, such as heart disease, type 2 diabetes, stroke, and cancer.

Defy The Effects of Aging: Get Your Antioxidants

A healthy diet is important at any age, but becomes critical, as you get older. The truth is that lifestyle diseases that stem from diet, and lack of physical activity are killing us.

The World Health Organization reports that lifestyle diseases account for a staggering 70% of all deaths and that more than ever before diet and lack of physical activity is driving these numbers in both industrial regions and developing countries.

Aging is an inevitable process; it will happen regardless of what you do. However, there are ways you can take the process in hand that offer a bit of a "slow down" of the process to avoid many preventable diseases that cause premature death. Wouldn't it be a lot better to reach old age healthy and full of vigor?

Making the right choices now will insure that you get older and at the same time feel great compared to uncle Joe who is laying in a hospital waiting to die.

What is the best place to start? By reading this and feeding your body with the foods it needs to optimize performance and health.

The Single Best Way To Slow Down Aging Consuming Antioxidants

You would have likely heard the word antioxidant but may not fully understand what it means or what it does within the body. Let's clear that up. See, as we age, every single day of our lives we are exposed to oxidation damage. It is simply a fact of life. Cells and DNA become worn out the longer they exist, and eventually, they are unable to replicate to 100%.

This is the process of aging. Stress from everyday life just compounds oxidative damage and can accelerate the aging process, exactly what we are trying to avoid.

Anti-Aging Benefits Of Anti-Oxidants

1. **Prevents you from getting UV Damage From The Sun -** damage from the sun can accelerate aging of the skin and result in cell mutations.

2. Boosts your Heart Health - Anti-oxidants can keep cholesterol levels within a normal range while clearing blood vessels. This promotes a normal heart rhythm.

3. Strengthens your Immune System - You become less susceptible to illnesses that sap away your health. Anti-oxidants make you more resistant to various types of cancer.

With that in mind, where are these antioxidants found?

Luckily, in a variety of veggies and fruits. For the best health, and graceful aging, consider getting more of the items below in your diet:

Berries

Berries are fruits with the highest antioxidant content. They positively boost your health. Think of blueberries, strawberries, and cranberries as ones you should be getting more of. I know they seem expensive, but their benefits far outweigh the costs. Though they are not to be consumed in mass amounts (due to sugar content) they do provide a massive dose of antioxidants with pro-inflammatory compounds that slow down hastened aging. They are also one of the lowest sugar fruits.

Cocoa

Cocoa has many more functions than making chocolate since it is actually a health food. Rich in polyphenols. One of which is epicatechin, cocoa has a myriad of health benefits including potent anti-inflammatory and antioxidant ability. Cocoa is superior in antioxidant profile when compared with green tea or even red wine.

Cruciferous Veggies

Cruciferous veggies include broccoli, Brussels sprouts, cabbage, cauliflower, collard **greens**, kale, kohlrabi, mustard, rutabaga, turnips, bok choy, and Chinese cabbage.

They are extremely rich in anti-oxidants and phytonutrients, cruciferous vegetables can help prevent cancer, improve blood lipid values and encourage the removal of waste from the body. Coupled with the fact that they're excellent free radical scavengers, cruciferous vegetables can and should be consumed daily.

Brightly Colored Veggies/ Fruits

Think of carrots, bell peppers and citrus, all foods that contain high number of bioactive compounds. In terms of carrots, they contain high levels of Beta-carotene, a type of vitamin A that has super potent antioxidant abilities.

Coupled with the high Vitamin C levels of bell peppers and citrus, these fruits and veggies provide a massive anti-aging effect in those who consume it. Tomatoes are also rich in lycopene, a rare antioxidant that is especially helpful to men's health.

Conclusion

Antioxidants are your best insurance against the rigors of aging. They help safeguard heart health, eye, and skin along with fortifying your immune system. Consuming a mix of both fruits and vegetables ensures you get the widest spectrum of phytonutrients available to prevent lifestyle diseases and maintain a healthy weight.

The Role Of Diet In Healthy Aging

There is one truth in life, you will eventually age into your golden years. Beyond that, there are no guarantees of course, but recent studies in nutrition science have shown that diet plays a key role in aging gracefully.

Whether you are looking at the bioactive compounds found in fruits and vegetables that promote healthy aging, flavonoids that reduce risks for oxidative stress or healthy fats that reduce the risk of cardiovascular disease, a healthy diet can have miraculous effects on how well you age and whether you will die prematurely from chronic disease.

What diet-related diseases am I at risk for as I age?

As you age, many things come into play when determining the risk factors for disease. According to the Center For Science In The Public Interest, the number one factor in determining your risk of death from disease is diet.

Diet can play an important role in the prevention and management of many age-related diseases including but not limited to:

- Heart disease

- Type 2 diabetes

- Obesity

- Stroke

- High blood pressure

- Osteoporosis

- Cancers (cervical, colon, gallbladder, kidney, liver, ovarian, uterine, postmenopausal breast cancer and others not related to smoking)

What are the best food choices to improve aging?

Choosing the best food for improving aging may be a matter of what you consider an improvement in your aging process. While it is true that pomegranates and blueberries contain free radical fighting antioxidants that may help fine lines and smooth your skin that may not be the most important thing for you to consider as you age.

The antioxidants contained in these foods can also help fight inflammation throughout the body which is going to be a far more important effect, than fighting wrinkles.

Including a wide variety of whole real food (and not processed junk) that provides with you a wide range of nutrients is your smartest choice, so you can cover the farthest range of disease preventing and health supporting benefits that sound nutrition provides. At the same time, it is important to limit or avoid junk and processed food that is typically lacking in nutrients, has unnecessary added fats and sugars and excess calories.

Is diet important for health and vitality in aging?

Diet can control many aspects of how you feel and how much energy you have. According to Web M.D., many foods give you a boost in energy and help you feel especially full of vitality even as you age. Nuts, lean meats, salmon, leafy greens, colorful vegetables and foods high in fiber.

This extra boost of energy may not seem important when you are young, but as you age, it becomes a key ingredient in maintaining a healthy and active lifestyle. Diet is one of the most important factors in maintaining health and vitality as you age.

Why is maintaining a healthy weight important as I get older?

Obesity is currently the number one cause of preventable death. About 1/3 of all adults are considered obese. These numbers present an epidemic level of the weight problem around the world. It highlights the need for vigilance in diet, and the need for regular exercise.

Obesity is also the culprit in many lifestyle diseases that prematurely kill thousands of people around the world. Overweight and obesity related health problems include coronary heart disease, high blood pressure, stroke, type 2diabetes, joint-related conditions, metabolic syndrome, sleep apnea, and the list goes on.

According to The National Heart Lung and Blood Institute, being overweight and obese along with age increases your risks for these diseases.

The last thing you want to do is give yourself a double dose of risk for these preventable and serious conditions as you grow older. Aging gracefully and living with vitality in your golden years means maintaining a healthy weight to reduce the risks of many preventable diseases and maintaining a high quality of life.

Is portion control important in aging?

Your body needs less food as you age because metabolism begins to naturaly slow as you get older. Most of us missed the memo, which is probably why we see a weight gain each year after age 50.

What does nutrient dense mean?

According to the National Institute of Health for Senior Health, nutrient dense foods are foods that have the most nutrients with the least calories. Therefore, food that is nutrient dense will provide you with a high amount of vitamins, minerals, lean proteins, complex carbohydrates and/or healthy fats with the least amount of calories.

For example, broccoli is nutrient dense, as a serving of it is very high in nutrients, but very low in calories. Conversely, a chocolate chip cookie is high in calories, but has very little nutrients so is not considered to be nutrient dense.

It is important to focus on nutrient dense foods as you age because every calorie counts, so food you eat needs to be of value. Additionally, people begin to see a drop in appetite as they get older and this means that they are not getting as many nutrients as they should because they are eating less food.

Eating nutrient dense food means that you are focused on the quality of the food rather than the quantity of the calories. This way you can ensure that your body will have everything it needs to keep functioning properly throughout your senior years.

What are the best heart health foods?

If you're looking at heart-healthy foods, you're going to want to incorporate things that reduce inflammation, maintain healthy cholesterol and blood pressure. All of these foods can help you reduce your risk for heart disease and live a longer and healthier life.

WebMD Recommends The Following Heart Healthy Foods:

- Fatty cold-water fish high in omega-3 fatty acids

- Berries that give you fiber and antioxidants

- Low-fat dairy containing calcium and vitamin D

- Whole-grain oats contain high amounts of fiber that have been shown to reduce bad (LDL) cholesterol

- Olive oil instead of butter because it contains heart healthy omega-3 fatty acids

- Dark chocolate for its antioxidants which helps keep bad cholesterol down

What are the best fats to support heart health?

Choosing healthy fats in the right amounts is key for heart health

- **Trans fats** – 0% or less than 2%

- **Saturated Fats** – less than 10% of total daily caloric intake

- **Monounsaturated Fats** – between 15% and 20% of total daily caloric intake

- **Polyunsaturated Fats** – between 5% and 10% of total daily caloric intake

BEST - UNSATURATED FATS - These include monounsaturated fats and polyunsaturated fats (omega-3 and omega-6 fatty acids). These are your healthiest choices for heart and brain health with the highest concentrations of omega-3 fatty acids found in cold-water fish (wild salmon, tuna, herring, and mackerel), nuts, and flaxseed.

In Moderation - **Saturated fats** - Saturated fats are typically found in dairy and meat products and are solid at room temperature. Saturated fats are associated with an increased risk of heart disease and should be moderated.

Avoid - **Trans fats** - Trans fats are heart killers and should be avoided at all costs. Most manufacturers have moved away from using trans fats in their foods because of risks associated with heart disease, though many packaged foods still have them. Check labels for hydrogenated oils.

What role do omega-3 fatty acids play in my health?

Omega-3's are monosaturated fats, which are responsible for many heart healthy effects within the body. They reduce inflammation, promote good HDL cholesterol, and keep you healthy as you age.

The University of Maryland reports that omega-3 fatty acids can help you reduce the risk and even reverse the effects of damage from the following conditions:

- High cholesterol
- High blood pressure
- Heart disease
- Diabetes
- Rheumatoid arthritis
- Lupus
- Osteoporosis
- Depression and bipolar disorder
- ADHD
- Cognitive decline
- Skin disorders
- IBS

Marine forms of omega-3 fatty acids offer **EPA and DHA** and are found in oily fish. Plant forms of omega-3 fatty acids offer **ALA** (alpha-linolenic acid), which is found in plant foods, oils, seeds and nuts. ALA is not nearly as potent as the marine sources of omega-3's EPA and DHA.

Good sources of EPA and DHA (Experts recommend two servings of fish each week)

- Mackerel
- Wild Caught Salmon
- Anchovies
- Bluefish
- Herring
- Sardines
- Sturgeon
- Lake trout
- Tuna

Good plant sources of ALA

Enjoy these healthy fats in moderation daily

- Walnuts and walnut oil
- Avocados and avocado oil
- Flaxseed and flaxseed oil
- Canola oil
- Soybean oil

Enjoy vegetables liberally

- Brussels sprouts
- Kale

- Mint
- Parsley
- Spinach
- Watercress

Does diet put women at higher risk for heart disease?

According to MedlinePlus, diet is the leading cause of heart disease for both men and women. If you are worried about heart disease, there are a few things that you can do to reduce your risk.

1. Eat five servings of fruit and vegetables every day

2. Eat whole grains

3. Choose lean healthy protein and cold water fish

4. Limit high intakes of saturated fats

5. Choose heart healthy monosaturated, polyunsaturated fats

6. Avoid trans fats completely

7. Sodium intake plays a significant role in heart disease, so limiting salt intake and cutting out processed foods that are high in salt can help reduce your risk for heart disease

What role do antioxidants play in the aging process?

There are many theories about why we age. One of the theories is oxidative stress caused by free radicals. Free radicals are atomic reactions within the mitochondria of cells that cause damage to cells within the body. This is known as oxidative damage. The free radical theory of aging is very technical but to sum it up free radicals cause inflammation and premature and accelerated aging.

It is thought that antioxidants can help reduce free radical damage to the body. Foods high in antioxidants have been shown to reduce risks for many age-related diseases like Alzheimer's, inflammatory diseases like arthritis, heart disease and others, which may actually be the result of oxidative damage due to free radicals. Live Science notes that our bodies can produce some antioxidants on their own but not in sufficient amounts to keep free radicals in check, making it important to eat foods that contain them, specifically fresh fruits and vegetables in all colors.

What foods reduce the risks for cancer?

The causes of many types of cancer are still generally unknown, though science does agree that antioxidants do play a key role in their prevention. Antioxidants are substances in food that provide protection to cells in the body from damage caused by free radicals that may lead to cancer. Numerous studies have shown that when antioxidants interact with free radicals they have the power to prevent some of this damage and therefore possibly reduce risks for the development of cancer.

WebMD's List Of Foods Highest In Antioxidants

- Purple, red, and blue grapes

- Small red, kidney and pinto beans

- Wild blueberry

- Cranberries

- Sweet potatoes

- Orange vegetables

- Artichoke (cooked)

- Blackberries

- Prune

- Raspberries

- Strawberries

- Red delicious, granny smith and gala apples

- Pecan

- Sweet cherries

- Black plums

- Russet potato (cooked)

- Black beans (dried)

- Plums

- Coffee is one of the American Institute for Cancer Research's most recommended foods for fighting cancer

What role does diet play in risks for stroke?

One of the most common age-related diseases and the most devastating is a stroke. Not only can a stroke change the course of your life but it will also effect everyone around you. Knowing the role that diet plays in reducing your risk for stroke can help you avoid this dangerous medical condition.

The Stroke Association recommends that your diet include:

- A variety of fruits and vegetables high in vitamins and minerals and fiber
- Unrefined whole grains
- Fish twice per week
- Avoiding foods high in saturated fat and cholesterol
- Avoiding refined sugars
- Limiting salt intake

What are key nutrients for the aging woman?

Women need to focus on specific nutritional needs as they age because they are at risk for specific age-related diseases, including osteoporosis from which they suffer at higher rates than men do. This means the intake of calcium and vitamin D is of utmost importance to keep bones strong and reduce risks for osteoporosis.

Menopause also presents the need for certain nutrients. While menopausal women need less iron, they do need an increase in vitamin B12 to reduce the risk of becoming anemic. Foods that are high in vitamin B12 include fish, shellfish, fortified cereals, dairy products, and eggs.

Discussing your body's changes with your physician may help you identify other nutritional deficiencies that you have after menopause.

What are key nutrients for the aging man?

Men and women are biologically different. That means that we need different things for our bodies to function properly. As men age, they need a host of different nutritional elements to help keep them healthy and active.

The Academy of Nutrition and Dietetics recommends the following for men to enjoy a healthy and active senior life.

Potassium: Older men need more potassium and they also need to decrease their salt intake. Potassium rich foods include fruits like bananas vegetables low-fat or fat-free milk and yogurt.

Omega 3 Fatty Acids: Men need a high amount of omega-3 fatty acids and healthy fats and at the same time they need to reduce their fat intake to 20 to 35% of their diet. Try swapping butter for heart-healthy canola oil or olive oil.

Other nutritional needs may exist, so it is important to talk with your doctor.

I love junk food, am I putting myself at risk?

Eating "bad foods" in moderation will not put you at risk for age-related and diet-related diseases (unless you have a pre-existing condition like diabetes or heart disease). The key is understanding what moderation is, specifically that it is splurging on occasion and in small amounts, allowing you to enjoy the occasional indulgence with little risk to your health.

Alternatively, if you indulge too much or worse yet all the time then yes you are most certainly putting yourself at very high risk for various lifestyle diseases, including heart disease, stroke, obesity, type 2 diabetes, and possibly premature death.

Is a plant diet good for healthy aging?

Plant-based diets are wonderful at any age. They are good for your waistline and provide you with ample vitamins, minerals, and antioxidants. There is only one concern when eating a plant-based diet, and that is that you are getting enough protein. Essential proteins are proteins that cannot be produced by your body.

Most complete essential proteins are only found in meat products. While plants may have a portion of a complete protein typically on their own, they do not have the entire protein chain. So when eating a plant-based diet, you need to make sure to eat certain foods.

Plant-based complete proteins:

- Quinoa

- Quorn

- Buckwheat

- Soy

Combined Proteins

- Beans and rice

- Ezekiel bread

- Seitan

- Hummus and pita

- Spirulina with grains or nuts

Assuming that you get your dietary allowance of protein, there is no reason not to enjoy a plant-based diet.

Can I reduce wrinkles with a good diet?

WebMD recommends many foods to help you reduce wrinkles. Here is a list of everything they recommend to keep your face looking younger.

- Eat more cold water fish for omega-3 fatty acids

- Eat more fruits and vegetables high in vitamin C that promotes collagen production

- Eat more protein that promotes collagen production

- Drink hot cocoa or eat at least 60% cacao chocolate that's key antioxidants have anti-aging properties for the skin

If you incorporate these foods into your diet, you can see a reduction in wrinkles because of the added benefits that these foods have in fighting age-related collagen reduction and elasticity loss in the skin.

What are the best foods for optimal energy in the older years?

As you age, your nutritional profile changes. The nutritional needs of a two-year-old are different from that of a 15-year-old. Someone in their 30s is not going to need the same amount of calories as a 15-year-old. An 80-year-old is going to have far different nutritional needs than a 30-year-old.

Key nutritional staples in the older population:

- **Lots of fruits and vegetables:** These are high-energy foods that offer you key nutrients to help the body function and perform at its best.

- **Increase protein intake:** 15 to 20% of your calories should come from protein. This will help you repair age related muscle loss.

- **Omega-3 fatty acids:** getting enough omega-3 fatty acids reduces your risk of heart disease, Alzheimer's and many other age-related degenerative diseases. Eat oily fish at least twice a week.

- **Calcium and vitamin D:** these two go hand-in-hand to help maintain strong bones and prevent osteoporosis, but you cannot absorb calcium without vitamin D, so you need to have both in adequate amounts. If you're not spending time out in the sun to get your vitamin

D, you need to take a supplement. Most calcium supplements are paired with vitamin D to help your body absorb the nutrient. Strong bones allow you to be more active in your older years.

Are there are any joint health-friendly foods?

Achy joints just seem to come with the territory of aging, most of this is thanks to the high prevalence of arthritis. Learning how to fight the aches and pains that can come with aging can help improve your quality of life. Joint pain can be debilitating and lead to inactivity, obesity, and has an impact on mental health. Luckily, diet can help improve joint pain. The Arthritis Foundation has listed many foods that will help you fight joint pain and inflammation.

- Fish for omega-3 fatty acids

- Turmeric the spice or in supplement form is an all-natural anti-inflammatory

- Swap butter for cooking oils high in omega-3 fatty acids, such as walnut oil

- Cherries have been shown to reduce the risk of gout and have anti-inflammatory effects, due to their red color

The arthritis foundation has a lot of good information for joint health and mobility. If you're suffering from joint pain they may be your best resource other than a good healthy diet.

What foods support bone health in women?

Building better bone health as you age is a top priority. The risk of falls combined with brittle bones caused by osteoporosis can create disaster and lead to hospitalization or worse. Knowing how to support bone health through nutrition can be the best way to prevent broken bones and fractures in your golden years.

The National Osteoporosis Foundation has published a list of wonderful foods that have either calcium or vitamin D to help you build strong, healthy bones. Remember your body has to have both calcium and vitamin D to absorb any amount of calcium. 30 minutes in the sun will give you enough vitamin D. You can get it from a diet with these foods that support bone health.

- Dairy products: Fortified with vitamin D

- Fatty fish like salmon: vitamin D

- Deep green vegetables: Vitamin D and calcium.

- Fortified foods like breakfast cereals, soy milk and juices give you calcium and vitamin D.

Make sure to ask your doctor about your levels of vitamin D, as blood tests can assess your levels and if you need supplements. For more information, visit The National Osteoporosis Foundation.

What are the best workout fuel foods for ages 50+?

It's best to stay active and healthy throughout your life to ensure that you lead a high-quality existence while you are on this planet. Learning how to properly fuel your workouts as you age can help you stay energetic through your workouts.

If you've stayed active and healthy up to age 50, your nutritional profile pre-workout probably won't change much. You still want to eat a small amount of carbohydrates 30 minutes to one hour before workout.

All of these are also going to give you bonus effects such as reducing the risk of heart disease and lowering your LDL-cholesterol. Eating after age 50 is all about reducing the risk of age-related disease, even before a workout.

- Whole-Grain Oats

- Bananas

- Apples

- Berries

- Beans

As I get older, I am concerned about my health, should I cut back sugar?

There are multiple reasons to be concerned about sugar intake no matter your age. As you get older age-related disease becomes an increasing concern. Since many of these age-related diseases can be linked to obesity, sugar intake should be monitored closely.

The American Heart Association suggests that men eat no more than 150 calories from added sugar a day and women eat no more than 100 calories from added sugar a day.

Some of the other reasons you will want to limit your intake of sugar is that it has been linked to inflammation in the body, it may cause heart disease, increased risk for type 2 diabetes, and it causes weight gain. Refined sugar is really at best a useless food and at worst a harmful indulgence with zero nutritional value.

Are there any ways to make vegetables more enjoyable?

If you're not used to eating a vegetable-rich diet, vegetables can taste bland and flavorless. Incorporating vegetables into your diet may be a slow process at first, but there are things that you can do to make them taste better.

1. Decrease your sugar and junk intake. High amounts of sugar and fat in the diet can make whole food taste flavorless. As you decrease your intake of junk food, you will begin to appreciate the taste of real food.

2. Roast vegetables with herbs and spices. Steamed bland vegetables tend to be tasteless! Try roasting your vegetables with some extra virgin olive oil and your favorite blend of salt-free spices and this should give you great tasting dishes.

3. Grill them on the barbecue! Barbecued vegetables are amazing, they are even better if you marinade them first. You can marinade vegetables just as you would marinade meat and it gives them an amazing flavor especially after being cooked over an open flame.

What are the best foods to boost my immunity?

Preventing illness as you age is one of the most important things you can do. Proper nutrition is one of the best ways to boost your immune system and build-up your illness protection response.

Immunity Boosting Foods:

1. **Yogurt** contains probiotics which can help balance natural bacteria in your digestive system to help you fight infection and illness

2. **Oats and barley** contain beta-glucans that give your body antimicrobial and antioxidant capabilities to help fight off influenza and other commonly contracted illnesses.

3. **Garlic** is one of the best foods for fighting infection and bacteria. Garlic is even known as an anti-parasitic food. To get the immune boosting effective garlic, you

need to eat one or two whole cloves of fresh raw garlic daily.

4. **Tea** can help you produce virus-fighting interferon. A Harvard study had people drink 5 cups of black tea every day for two weeks, and they had 10 times more interferon in their blood than those who drink a placebo. It really is amazing that tea can have this much of an effect on your body.

There are even more foods that will help give your body and immune boost but remember following a healthy diet year-round with a high intake of fresh vegetables is going to be your best bet for leading a healthy life.

24 Anti-Aging Diet Tips

Whether you're 20 or 60, it's never too late for a healthy lifestyle in which diet is key to enjoying good health and a longer life. Growing old is inevitable, you can't escape from it but by making smarter dietary choices you can add years to your life.

Olive oil is rich in powerful antioxidants that significantly reduce risks for heart disease even in those at higher risk. Olives provide great amounts of polyphenols and other phytonutrients that help protect your DNA and keep you looking and feeling younger.

Fiber helps moderate your weight, decreasing your chances of obesity and all its many complications that make you sicker as you age.

Black currants contain anthocyanosises, which helps protect your eyesight and vitamin C that keeps your skin taut and wrinkle-free.

Pineapples are rich in manganese that is essential for activating an enzyme called prolinase that supports production of collagen for more youthful radiant skin.

Vegetables, legumes, fruits, and whole grains provide a wonderful supply of dietary fiber that keeps cholesterol levels in check.

Reduce or better yet eliminate processed and junk food from your diet, eat clean, whole food created by nature and you will enjoy much better health in your older years.

The risk for osteoporosis increases as the years pile on, one you hit 50 increase calcium intake to 1200 mg daily.

Turmeric contains curcumin that helps prevent the shortening of telomeres, the end caps of DNA, which leads to aging and degenerative diseases.

The nutrients found in tomatoes are linked to prevention of the sticking together of blood platelets in the arteries, which helps reduce risks for stroke and heart attack. Cooking tomatoes doubles their lycopene power and maximizes their anti-aging effects.

Cucumbers with an unwaxed peel offer silica to boost collagen production and reduce wrinkles for younger looking skin.

Tofu, soymilk, and other soy foods are rich in isoflavones to keep skin taut and youthful by preserving collagen and preventing the breakdown of collagen in aging.

One of the best-known choices in fish for its anti-aging effects is cod, which contains selenium that protects the skin from sun damage and skin cancer.

2 or 3 Brazil nuts is equivalent to the daily value of selenium, a powerful antioxidant that plays a critical role in DNA synthesis.

Tuna, wild salmon, mackerel, sardines, anchovies, and trout are great sources of omega-3 fatty acids that support healthy cholesterol and heart health.

Pumpkin seeds contain high levels of zinc, which helps reduce inflammation inside the body.

Sesame seeds are high in calcium, iron, magnesium, phosphorous and fiber, key nutrients for healthy aging.

Blueberries are low calorie fruits loaded with antioxidants to fight free radicals that can damage cells in the body and cause wrinkles.

Blueberries contain compounds that help prevent inflammation and oxidative damage, both of which are linked to age-related memory and motor function issues.

Cherries are rich in the anti-cancer agent known as queritrin.

Strawberries contain natural anti-inflammatory agents called phytonutrients that protect your heart and vitamin C that helps prevent wrinkles and dryness of the skin.

The Quest For Younger Looking Healthy Skin

We all want smooth skin that glows with radiance and youth, and there is a long line of anti-aging beauty products that promise just that. However, did you ever stop to notice that these long lines of cosmetic products are infused with food products? And that they're usually the most expensive?

This makes you wonder if it wouldn't be better to nourish our skin from the inside out by eating the foods that give it the most benefits instead of just applying it to the skin's surface?

"Nutrition plays an important part in limiting the aging process and helping to protect against damage from UV rays, the number one cause of lines and wrinkles," says Adam Friedman, M.D., director of dermatologic research at Albert Einstein College of Medicine in New York City.

The key to aging gracefully is eating healthy

This fact is not just skin deep; sticking to a healthy diet also helps fight off diseases, prevents weight gain and type diabetes, as well as decreases our risk of cancer. A lot of research has been carried out on how certain nutrients help protect our bodies from harmful environmental factors, and prevent oxidative stress that causes premature and accelerated aging of the skin.

Proper nutrition is also key in keeping the skin's cells hydrated and functioning at their optimal levels.

Foods Rich In Vitamin C

Vitamin C is one of the best-known antioxidants to protect the skin from free radicals, which are unstable molecules and atoms that wreak havoc on our cells and cause oxidative stress that accelerates aging.

Vitamin C is found in a variety of foods:

- Bell peppers

- Oranges

- Lemons

- Guava

- Limes

- Berries

- Grapefruits

- Broccoli

- Berries

- Sweet potatoes

These foods are more than able to provide you with your daily intake, which can range from 65 - 90 mg per day. One cup of strawberries will provide you with roughly 150% of the daily recommended amount of vitamin C. Eating a large orange will also provide you with a good amount of vitamin C, as well as hydrate your skin and keep it supple since oranges are full of water.

Studies show that those who regularly incorporate foods rich in vitamin C into their diets reduce their risk of wrinkles by 36%.

Their skin also showed signs of being well hydrated, which means radiant, younger-looking skin. Vitamin C also protects the skin against UV radiation.

To make sure your body is getting the most of your vitamin C intake, combine it with foods that contain vitamin E, which protects the skin from the sun and other inflammatory agents.

Lean Protein

As we age, collagen and other proteins in our skin break down making the skin slump into itself, which creates fine lines and wrinkles. Eating protein helps your skin rebuild collagen and elastin, which work together to keep skin taut, supple and smooth in texture.

"Protein provides the building blocks of collagen," says F. William Danby, M.D., adjunct assistant professor of surgery (dermatology) at Dartmouth Medical School.

- Eggs are a great source of protein since they are a perfect protein containing all essential amino acids that help protect the skin against wrinkles, lysine, proline, and glycine.

- Eggs also contain other healthy nutrients such as vitamin A, E, selenium, and iron all of which play a role in collagen formation.

You can also choose 2 to 4-ounce servings of skinless chicken breasts, fish, pork or beef two or three times a week. Just remember when you're cooking beef to flip it often to prevent it from crisping and charring since that will undo all of its the anti-aging properties.

Omega-3 Fatty Acids

We've all heard how fish is packed with omega-3 fatty acids, but what exactly does that mean? Omega-3s (monosaturated) are the good type of fats, along with omega-6 (polyunsaturated) that help plump up skin cells, making them well hydrated, less wrinkly and more protected against sun damage which reduces the risk of skin cancer.

They basically moisturize the skin from the inside out as well as protect it from harmful UV rays. They're also very good for your heart health.

- Eating **two 6-ounce servings of fatty fish weekly** that are rich in omega-3, which contain EPA and DHA is essential. There are plenty to choose from, such as mackerel, herring, lake trout, and sardines. However, two of the best-known fish that are packed with omega-3 are tuna and wild salmon.

- **Walnuts, flaxseeds, avocados, pumpkin seeds, and olive oil** are all excellent sources of omega-3.

Salmon

The reason why salmon - especially wild salmon - really stands out is that besides its omega-3 content, it contains a **powerful antioxidant known as astaxanthin**. This carotenoid gives it its signature pink color, but besides making it look gorgeous, this antioxidant **helps wipe out harmful free radicals and reduces the risk of skin cancer.**

Nuts

Like olive oil, nuts in general are a great source of unsaturated fats, vitamins, minerals, and antioxidants. Eating a handful of mixed nuts for an afternoon snack provides you with a healthy portion of omega-3 fatty acids to nourish your skin, as well as anti-inflammatory **properties to** help treat and prevent skin conditions like eczema, psoriasis, and acne.

- Walnuts are known for having the highest levels of omega-3s

- Almonds are best known for their high vitamin E content

- Brazil nuts are chock-full of selenium. They're also a great source of vitamin E, which makes them the ideal choice for slowing down the aging process.

- Other types of nuts, like hazelnuts, peanuts and pistachios, are also good for your health when eaten in moderation.

Avocados

Avocados contain vitamin E, C and B-complex that help protect and nourish the skin and keep it supple.

Avocados also contain monounsaturated fat, a healthy fat, which helps the body absorb the vitamins and nutrients your skin needs, as well as keep it well hydrated.

Olive Oil

Olive oil is known to contain high levels of monounsaturated fats. Olive oil can lower the risk of heart disease and cancer. It also has polyphenols and potent antioxidants that help keep you wrinkle-free. Olive oil is also wonderful when used topically to moisture and nourish the skin.

Whole Grains

Whole grains contain the mineral selenium, which plays a major role in protection against the damage caused by UV radiation. Eating 3 to 4 servings daily of the following will provide you with your fair share of selenium, while at the same time, managing your weight:

- **Brown rice** contains high levels of fiber, potassium, proteins, magnesium, thiamine, and calcium

- **Barley** is an excellent source of fiber, selenium, copper, phosphorus, magnesium, niacin. Moreover, it works at decreasing cholesterol levels in the blood and reducing the risk of heart disease

- **Steel Cut Or Rolled Oats** are a good example of complex carbohydrates that are low on the glycemic index, which means they're good for keeping blood sugar levels in check.

- Oats also have a natural plant chemical that helps soothes irritated skin and wards off skin cell damage. They are also a good source of zinc. Always choose cut or rolled whole grain oats, and not instant oatmeal products to get the most nutritional value.

- **Buckwheat** is an excellent source of a bioflavonoid that helps the body utilizes vitamin C called rutin. Rutin provides the skin with elasticity and firmness and helps keep collagen levels in check.

- **Wheat germ** has nutrients that help keep the skin smooth and reduce the appearance of wrinkles. It's a great source of vitamin E that is essential for maintaining healthy-looking skin. It contains vitamin B6, coenzyme Q10 and protein. Make sure your store it in a sealed container away from the sun because it goes rancid fast due to its unsaturated fat content.

Vibrant Colorful Produce

Carotenoids are what make up the colors you see in fruits and vegetables, herbs and spices, and even salmon. They are also antioxidants that wipe out free radicals and help fight against inflammations and diseases. They also help with the production of collagen, hydrating your skin from the inside out and help protect against the damage caused by harmful UV rays.

Sweet Potatoes

These delicious vegetables can help delay the signs of aging because they contain the carotenoid, beta-carotene. They are also a great source of vitamin C.

The best part about eating sweet potatoes is that studies show that they help produce HA (hyaluronic acid) which helps keep the skin supple and smooth and is mainly produced by the body.

Unfortunately, the body's ability to produce this acid decreases with age but adding sweet potatoes to your diet can help keep the levels of HA at a steady level.

Grapes

The skin of grapes contains polyphenols called resveratrol, which act like antioxidants and help fight inflammation. Resveratrol reduces the damage from UV rays. Some studies also show that it may slow down the aging process.

Blueberries

If you're looking for something to add to your diet that has major benefits bundled together, look no further. Blueberries, as well as raspberries, contain **antioxidants, probiotics, anthocyanins, vitamins, polyphenols, and flavonoids. They truly are the whole package.**

Moreover, they help the skin regenerate new cells, which, slows the aging process. They also fight off free radicals while helping replenish the skin cells natural plumpness and elasticity.

Carrots

One of the best sources of beta-carotene, carrots are great at protecting the skin against free radicals and damage from sun exposure. They also contain a great deal of nutrients and vitamins, including vitamin C.

Tomatoes

Best known for containing lycopene, which helps wipe out the harmful effects of UV rays, tomatoes are a great addition to your diet. Found also in watermelon, pink grapefruit, carrots, guava and red pepper, lycopene also boosts the vascular system, giving your cheeks a nice rosy color.

Lycopene is better absorbed by the body when it's in the form of processed tomato products, such as tomato paste, pasta sauce, and ketchup, and when tomatoes are cooked.

When eaten with foods containing beta-carotene, it's absorbed even more by the body, which is lucky for us because tomatoes also contain beta-carotene. Tomatoes also help reduce the appearance of fine lines and wrinkles, mainly because they contain vitamin C as well which helps produce collagen and plump up skin cells.

Apples

Besides keeping the doctor away, apples also are great at keeping wrinkles away. They contain vitamin C, the powerful antioxidant quercetin, flavonoids and are also a great source of fiber.

Celery

Celery contains beta-carotene, and vitamins E and C. All these work at reducing the presence of wrinkles by hydrating the skin from the inside out and keep it supple and firm.

Onions

Also containing quercetin, onions are a great health booster and a wonderful addition to any diet. Onions contain sulfur, which help keep the skin supple, smooth and protected from harmful external factors.

Leafy Green Vegetables

Spinach

A great source of beta-carotene, vitamins E, and C, as well as several other nutrients that help keep wrinkles at bay. It also has high levels of glutathione, which is a powerful antioxidant that helps, fight off inflammation and harmful free radicals that accelerate aging, including that which affects the skin and its appearance.

Broccoli

Broccoli contains beta-carotene, vitamin C and the co-enzyme Q10 - all healthy boosters to slow down the aging process and provide you with essential health benefits.

Brussels sprouts

If you gave your mother a hard time eating your Brussel sprouts, now is the time to call and apologize. These cute vegetables contain wrinkle-fighting agents such as vitamins C and A, as well as folate. Vitamin C helps with the production of collagen, while the last two helps protect your skin against sun damage.

Soy Foods

Soy foods are typically rich in isoflavones, which are potent wrinkle-fighting agents because they help prevent the deterioration of collagen. Soybeans are an excellent source of protein, very similar to eggs. Tofu also helps safeguard collagen levels in the skin.

Honey

Ask any beautician and they'll tell you honey is one of the best things you can put on your face for a clean and glowing complexion. It also does wonders for your skin from the inside out. Honey is antiviral, antibacterial, and a powerful antioxidant; it helps fight inflammation, wipes out free radicals, and plumps up skin cells to keep your skin supple and soft.

Yogurt

Foods packed with probiotics can help treat and prevent inflammations and irritations from the inside, which can clear skin problems such as eczema, redness of the skin, psoriasis, and acne. You can also use it as a facemask - the lactic acid found in yogurt will tighten pores and help eliminate dead skin cells. It can also reduce wrinkles, fine lines, blemishes as well as act as a great moisturizer for the skin.

Best Drinks For Healthy Skin

Water

One of the best ways to have soft, smooth, youthful skin is by regularly drinking water. Water hydrates helping to keep the skin well moisturized, something that is lost as a normal part of the aging process. Water also helps lower blood pressure levels and protects joints and organs. It also helps minimize the risk of dementia because it keeps brain cells functioning properly and increases your concentration span and ability to focus.

Green Tea

When you drink green tea, especially if you seep loose tea leaves for about 5 minutes, then you're on your way to preventing wrinkles via the catechins found in green tea. Catechins are compounds that help cells grow and function properly. They also contain antioxidant properties, which help clear away free radicals that harm the skin due to sun exposure.

Green tea also contains polyphenols that help reduce the risk of non-melanoma skin cancer as well as help replenish skin cells to keep them hydrated and healthy.

Coffee

Even though caffeine is known to be a diuretic that can make you excrete precious fluids and drain your body of its moisture. It ends up leaving your skin looking dull and haggard.

Coffee in moderation (2 to 3 cups daily) it has many benefits including that it has been proven to reduce your risk of skin cancer by nearly 10%. Drinking decaf doesn't offer the same protection.

Cocoa

As teenagers, we were warned of what chocolate can do to our skin. However, the surprising news is that nothing has been proven to tie quality dark cacao to skin problems.

The truth is cocoa may be very good for your skin and that is probably because of a certain type of flavonoid called epicatechin which increases the flow of nutrients, oxygen supply, and blood to the surface of the skin - all important elements for healthy, supple skin. Epicatechin can also be found in tea and red wine.

Will Supplements Do The Trick?

While there are numerous ways to get the nutrients, your body needs from pills or special drinks, it's still considered expensive and a secondary option to getting all of your skin-enhancing minerals and vitamins naturally from food.

All the antioxidants, essential fatty acids, and your complete dose of nutrients can be easily obtained from the diet and is really the best way.

Key Tips To Look And Feel Younger

To look and feel younger, here are a few general tips:

- Choose foods that are naturally chock-full of nutrients and antioxidants which help protect our cells and their DNA from harmful factors that can hamper the production of our skin's main supporting fabric, collagen.

- Vary your diet so you and your body get a vast variety of essential nutrients, such as vitamins, minerals, and antioxidants.

- Remember that a healthy lifestyle goes hand in hand with a healthy diet and everything you do affects the health and appearance of your skin:

  - Sleep well

  - exercise regularly

  - Reduce stress

- be cautious when you're spending time in the sun and always wear sunscreen

- Drink alcohol in moderation

- Don't smoke cigarettes

Thoughts

Many factors and variables go into the aging process, but you have many options in determining how well you will age. If eating a healthy diet can improve how well your skin will age, why not do it?

Especially if it'll also benefit you in all other aspects, such as your weight, cholesterol, blood pressure, diabetes, osteoporosis and many other lifestyle diseases that afflict the aging and which are preventable.

By choosing healthy nutrient dense foods, you'll start noticing a difference in how your face glows and how soft it feels every time you look in the mirror.

Eating ample amounts of essential nutrients can delay the aging process, reduce risks for skin cancer, improve the condition of your skin, help reduce dark spots and eliminate fine lines.

The best part? With a few tweaks here and there, you've got yourself a delicious array of colorful, tasty dishes and drinks to last a lifetime.

Anti Aging Foods

These 30 anti-aging foods will provide you with the nutrients and minerals your body needs in order to remain robust, energetic, vital and most of all, young. Add these to your diet and you'll feel the difference fast.

When studies were carried out by the Seven Countries Study several decades ago, they found out that the reason behind the low rates of cancer and heart disease of those living in Crete were the monounsaturated fats found in olive oil.

It's widely-known that one of the key components of the Mediterranean diet is olive oil.
Since then, many studies have been carried out proving that olive oil is rich in powerful antioxidants called polyphenols that help ward off diseases largely related to aging, such as heart diseases and type-2 diabetes.

Polyphenols also contain potent anti-inflammatory agents, which help control cholesterol levels among other health benefits. Besides cooking with it and adding it to your salad, you can also use it as a natural moisturizer on your skin, as it can help prevent and reduce wrinkles due to its antioxidant content.

Olives

Since olive oil has such considerable health benefits, it is understood that its source would do the same. Olives are cute little salty fruits that provide great amounts of polyphenols and other phytonutrients that help protect your DNA and keep you looking and feeling younger. Make sure you eat the ones with the pits since removing the pits reduces the amount of phytonutrients found in each olive.

Fiber

Fiber is great at overseeing that your digestive system is running smoothly, helps ease constipation and keeps everything flowing smoothly. Fiber also helps moderate your weight, decreasing your chances of obesity. It also controls blood sugar levels and lowers your risk of diabetes.

Vegetables and whole grains provide a wonderful supply of dietary fiber, which also monitors your blood pressure, keeps your cholesterol levels in check, and lowers risks of inflammation.

Steel cut oats are high in soluble fiber, which reduces bad LDL cholesterol. Rich in healthier complex carbohydrates, whole oatmeal is one of the best-known comfort foods that boosts the release of serotonin, a feel-good hormone in the brain.

Yogurt

Yogurt is of course known for its high levels of calcium, which helps protect bones from osteoporosis. Yogurt also has the good type of bacteria, which helps the digestive system do its job, as it should. Yogurt has protein as well, for cell health and support of muscle, which naturally declines with age.

Choose yogurt that is fortified with vitamin D in order to get the most benefit out of the calcium, since vitamin D is needed for calcium absorption.

Turmeric

Turmeric's yellow pigment curcumin helps prevent telomeres from shortening. These are the end caps of our DNA and when shortened are a leading cause in aging and degenerative diseases. The shorter they get, the more cellular aging takes place, as well as increased risks for heart disease, cancer, and Alzheimer's disease.

Cold Water Fish & Seafood

Cold water oily fish such as **tuna, wild salmon, mackerel, sardines, anchovies,** and **trout** are great sources of omega-3 fatty acids.

Omega-3 Fatty Acids offer key health benefits in aging

- Reduction in elevated blood triglyceride levels

- Healthy cholesterol and heart health

- Can alleviate joint pain and stiffness that results from rheumatoid arthritis

- Limited research suggests that omega-3 fatty acids may help protect against dementia conditions, including Alzheimer's disease and may also prevent age related gradual memory loss linked to aging. These studies are limited and so not conclusive, but they are promising.

- Proven to help keep your skin looking radiant and help prevent skin cancer

- One type of omega-3 fatty acids found in seafood, EPA (eicosapentaenoic acid), is known for its ability to protect and maintain the fibrous protein that makes your skin taut, and firm in your youth called collagen. EPA also repairs damage caused by the sun's harmful rays.

- Omega-3s reduce low-grade inflammation from all the wear and tear on our bodies from stress, lack of sleep, unhealthy eating, and exposure to chemicals. We exhaust our immune system just cleaning up all that havoc wreaked on our bodies, which eventually accelerates the aging of our brains.

One of the best-known choices in fish for its anti-aging effects is **cod,** which contains selenium that protects the skin from sun damage and skin cancer by decreasing inflammatory compounds that can lead to tumor growth.

Seafood is also a wonderful source of protein, which helps build and sustain your muscles, and boosts your energy levels.

Oysters are rich in **zinc,** which is largely responsible for protein synthesis as well as the formation of collagen for younger looking skin.

Dark Chocolate

Eating dark chocolate drink will help curb your sweet tooth and is rich in flavonoids, which benefit the body by increasing blood flow to the skin. Flavonoids also absorb UV radiation, which means they protect your skin from the damaging effects of the sun.

They are also one of the best ways to main healthy functioning of blood vessels, which lowers your risk of high blood pressure, type 2 diabetes, dementia, and even kidney disease. One- or two-ounce squares daily are quite enough to avoid weight gain, as chocolate is high in calories.

Nuts

Studies show that those who eat nuts regularly live an average of 2 ½ years longer than those who do not. Nuts give you heathy unsaturated fats and omega-3s. They also have a vast variety of essential vitamins, fiber, protein, minerals, and phytochemicals, including antioxidants.

A handful of **almonds**, roughly about 23, contain 34% of your daily nutritional value of vitamin E, which helps with anti-inflammatory process in the body. It also helps bolster the immune system and protects cells from the damaging effects of free radicals. Vitamin E is an antioxidant not made naturally by the body but can only be obtained from food.

Just two or three South American **Brazil nuts** provides the daily recommended value of selenium, a powerful antioxidant that plays a critical role in DNA synthesis. It also helps protect the body from oxidative damage that accelerates aging and promotes disease and infection. These mineral repairs cell damage and slows down the skin's aging process, and its concentrations in the body begin to dwindle with age so obtaining it from food is important.

Eating a 1-ounce serving of nuts (one handful) 5 days a week is optimal to get their maximum benefit, you do not want to overdo it, as nuts are high in calories.

Seeds

Whether you prefer **pumpkin, sunflower,** or **flaxseeds,** if you're including them in your diet, you're on the right track. Seeds are rich in nutrients, plant proteins, and healthy fats. You can eat them on their own, or as snack bars, in your cereal, or on top of salads or desserts.

Sunflower seeds contain lignin phytoestrogens, which give a boost to your skin's lipid barrier and prevent the breakdown of collagen, keeping your skin radiant and glowing.

Pumpkin seeds contain high levels of zinc, which helps reduce inflammation inside the body that may accelerate aging. For an afternoon snack, munch on ¼ cup of unshelled pumpkin seeds to get your daily dose of zinc.

Sesame seeds are high in calcium, fiber and iron as well as other key minerals such as magnesium, and phosphorous. Tahini, made from sesame seeds, can be used as a base for a Vinaigrette, or seeds can be sprinkled on salads, fish, chicken or inside sandwiches.

Blueberries

Blueberries are highly nutrient rich fruits that should be enjoyed every day. These delicious low calorie fruits are loaded with antioxidants to fight free radicals that can damage cells in the body and cause wrinkles.

Blueberries contain compounds that help prevent inflammation and oxidative damage, both of which are linked to age-related memory and motor function issues. A study published by Tufts University reports that the blue color of blueberries results from anthocyanins, which help prevent oxidative stress, one of the key components of unhealthy aging. Anthocyanins also promote the production of dopamine in the brain helping to keep memory function healthy and boost positive mood.

Blueberries have more antioxidants than almost any other fruit. These antioxidants help protect skin cells against harmful UV-related damage from sun exposure, pollution and stress. Vitamin C keeps your skin looking youthful and wrinkle-free.

Here are more benefits of blueberries:

- Reduce risks of cancer

- <u>Reduce cholesterol levels</u>

- Reduce risks of heart disease and stroke

- May reduce risks of neurological diseases

- Brain and memory health

- Support immune system health

- Improve urinary tract health

- Improve vision and eye health

Other Berries

- **Black raspberries** are powerful cancer fighters. They're harder to find fresh, so it's more likely you'll find them in the frozen section.

- **<u>Cherries</u>** are rich in the anti-cancer agent known as quercitrin.

- **Strawberries** contain natural anti-inflammatory agents called phytonutrients that protect your heart in addition to having cancer-fighting properties. They also contain large amounts of vitamin C, which helps prevent wrinkles and dryness of the skin, both symptoms of aging, one cup of strawberries delivers about 150% of the daily recommended amount.

- **Blackberries** help prevent chronic diseases and reduce the risk of cancer since they contain a healthy dose of antioxidants, ellagic acid, as well as vitamins C and E.

- **Cranberries** are chock-full of polyphenols, a powerful antioxidant. Polyphenols may help reduce the risk of cancer, as well as inhibit the growth of cancer cells, and reduce inflammation from gum disease and stomach ulcers.

- **Acai berries** contain antioxidants and are capable of destroying cultured human cancer cells. They can be mainly found in Brazil.

Fresh Raw Garlic

Garlic is known as the triple-threat since it has antibacterial, antiviral, and antifungal properties mainly due to the antioxidant, allicin, which is what gives garlic its potent taste and smell.

It protects the body from several types of cancer, is known to improve blood flow by relaxing blood vessels, may help prevent plaque from building up in the arteries, lower cholesterol, and help regulate blood pressure.

Once it's been cut, garlic tends to lose its potency within one hour. So the best way to eat it is to take freshly chopped or pressed garlic, wait a few minutes so you get the maximum benefits then eat it, preferably by swallowing it whole, rather than chewing it. Powdered or dried garlic doesn't have the same effect as fresh garlic does.

Leafy Greens

Leafy greens such as **spinach, kale, turnip greens, collard greens**, and **romaine lettuce**, are nutrient dense power vegetables, true gifts from nature.

Kale is truly a nutrition powerhouse!

- It is an *excellent* source of antioxidants, vitamin K1, vitamin C, beta carotene (converted in the body to vitamin A), copper and manganese

- It is a *very good* source of vitamin B6, vitamin E, vitamin B2, calcium, fiber and potassium

- It is a *good* source of iron, magnesium vitamin B1, omega-3 fats, phosphorus, protein, folate, and vitamin B3

Kale can do so much for your body, and many of its benefits are directly related to healthier aging:

- Prevents oxidative stress that accelerates aging

- Protects from damage caused by free radicals

- Immune system health

- Healthy blood pressure

- Healthy blood clotting

- Reduced risk for cancer

- Skin health

- Healthy cholesterol for heart health

- Contains lutein and zeaxanthin, which numerous studies have shown to greatly reduce risks for age related macular degeneration and cataracts, two of the most common eye disorders in older people

Romaine lettuce is high in beta-carotene, which turns into vitamin A in the body and supports skin health by increasing new skin cell growth.

Spinach is also packed with antioxidants shown in studies to fight cancer, like beta-carotene, vitamin C, and sulforaphane. Vitamin C also keeps your hair and skin looking shiny and smooth, while minimizing dryness.

Spinach also contains folate, which helps preserve short-term memory. Folate also reduces the risk of heart disease and cancer since it slows down low-grade inflammations caused by the wear and tear of DNA. Spinach also has the ability to destroy dangerous free radicals that wreak havoc on our cells.

Some leafy greens, like collard greens, salad greens, kale and **spinach**, contain the all-important vitamin K1, which offers numerous benefits:

- Plays a major role in keeping veins healthy and relaxed, and helps prevent varicose veins

- Important for maintaining strong bones

- Helps regulate blood sugar levels

- Healthy blood clotting

- Heart health

- May protect from Alzheimer's disease

- Reduced risks of certain cancers, such as lung and liver cancer

Caution: Vitamin K1 interferes with blood thinner medications, ask your doctor.

Broccoli

Broccoli is a dark green vegetable that is part of the cruciferous family. While all cruciferous vegetables are highly health promoting, broccoli contains the most isothiocyanates (organosulfur compounds), of all the vegetables in this family.

- Isothiocyanates promote the release of cancer-fighting genes and decreasing those that promote their propagation.

- Studies have found that eating ample amounts of cruciferous vegetables is linked to lower risks of lung and colon cancer, due to their high content of sulforaphane, a compound within the isothiocyanate group.

- Folate is another important vitamin provided by broccoli that is believed to decrease the risk of breast cancer in women.

- Vitamin K in broccoli supports bone health. The high amounts of vitamin C in this wonderful vegetable promotes youthful skin by enhancing collagen production lost due to aging and is a key antioxidant for preventing damage caused by free radicals.

- Broccoli is also high in fiber and the Department of Internal Medicine and Nutritional Sciences Program at the University of Kentucky confirms that a high fiber diet significantly lowers risk factors for chronic diseases, which are associated with aging, including heart disease, type 2 diabetes, stroke, and digestive disorders.

Other Cruciferous Vegetables:

- Arugula
- Bok choi
- Broccoli rabe
- Brussels sprout
- Cabbage

- Cauliflower
- Chinese broccoli
- Chinese cabbage
- Collard greens
- Daikon
- Horseradish
- Kale
- Kohlrabi
- – seeds and leaves
- Pak choi
- Radish
- Rutabaga
- Wasabi
- Watercress

Swiss Chard

Swiss chard is a great anti-aging vegetable choice providing you with chlorophyll, a nutrient that is believed to block the effects of chemicals that cause cancer. It is very low in calories and nutrient dense, so can be enjoyed liberally every single day.

One cup of Swiss chard gives a day's worth of vitamin K and beta-carotene for healthy bones, and eyes. The potassium in this dark leafy green helps to lower blood pressure, while magnesium and alpha-lipoic acid promote healthy blood sugar and insulin levels.

Tomatoes

Tomatoes get their gorgeous red color from lycopene, a pigment that helps keep your skin smooth and glowing. It also protects the skin from harmful UV radiations and helps prevent wrinkles.

Since lycopene is a powerful antioxidant, it is advised for heart health, strong bones, and possible cancer prevention.

Lycopene can help to lower cholesterol and triglyceride levels in the blood.

The nutrients found in tomatoes are linked to prevention of the sticking together of blood platelets in the arteries, which helps reduce risks for stroke and heart attack.

Cooking tomatoes doubles their lycopene power and maximizes their anti-aging effects.

Other foods that contain lycopene:

- Pink Grapefruit
- Carrots
- Watermelon
- Guava
- Red Peppers

Watermelon

Watermelon is a source of lycopene, which protects the skin from UV rays. Packed with lycopene, watermelon acts as a natural protector from the harmful effects of ultraviolet rays that damage and ages the skin and creates sunspots. Watermelon is also packed with water to help hydrate and plump your skin for all-natural anti-aging.

Cucumbers

This salad favorite is great for skin. Cucumbers have the highest water content of any food.

Cucumbers with an unwaxed peel offer silica to boost collagen production and reduce wrinkles for younger looking skin.

Soy Foods

Soy provides phytoestrogens, which are compounds that behave like estrogen and have been related to a decrease in cardiovascular disease and bone loss. Phytoestrogens mimic estrogen the female hormone that is depleted during menopause, making soy foods a possible option to hormone replacement therapy (HRT) for menopausal women suffering from symptoms.

Tofu, as well as other types of soy food, such as **edamame** and **soymilk**, is rich in isoflavones, which help keep your skin taut and youthful by preserving collagen in skin cells, and preventing the breakdown of collagen, which happens as we age.

Guava

This exotic fruit is packed with vitamin C, which boosts collagen production for smooth, youthful-looking skin. To get your dose of vitamin C, eat 2 cups of guava weekly.

Bell Peppers

Bell peppers have high amounts of vitamin C, a potent antioxidant, which may prevent certain types of cancers and cardiovascular disease.

They go great with everything, on the grill, in your stir-fry and in stews. Even when eaten raw as snacks with dips or in salads, they provide 158% of the daily value of vitamin C, which plays a great role in the healing of wounds, in fighting off infections and bolstering the functioning of the immune system and skin health.

Oranges

Oranges are also wonderful sources of vitamin C, which helps boost the immune system and builds collagen, which makes your skin more supple and younger-looking.

Blood Oranges

Blood oranges are very delicious and contain anthocyanins, which are antioxidants that combat free-radical damage and UV rays.

Black Currants

Black currant contains a compound called anthocyanosises, which helps protect your eyesight and improves vision. On top of that, black currant contains triple the amount of vitamin C found in oranges, which helps boost your immune system and keep your skin taut and wrinkle-free.

Pineapples

These juicy fruits are rich in manganese, which is essential for activating a certain enzyme called prolinase. This enzyme provides the amino acids needed for the formation of collagen in the skin, providing you with healthy, youthful, radiant skin.

Concord Grapes

Concord grapes are known for their dark purple skin and seeds, which are full of polyphenols, a compound proven to boost your brain power, keeping you sharp and alert.

They also bolster your arteries, reducing the risk of heart disease while increasing blood flow to the brain.

Since these grapes are harvested for a few short weeks during the fall, finding them fresh is very difficult, so opt for drinking 100% pure grape juice instead to get all the benefits of these potent fruits.

Mushrooms

Many studies have been carried out on the healing powers of mushrooms.

- They can reduce and prevent inflammation

- Help fight cancer

- Boost the immune system

- Detoxify the body naturally

- Protect the heart

- Mushrooms also provide B vitamins, which are crucial for turning your food into sustainable energy and promoting healthy metabolism

- Mushrooms are the only plant food that contains vitamin D, which helps the body absorb calcium and supports strong bones.

- A great bonus is the type of fiber found in mushrooms, called beta-glucan, which helps with weight management. Additionally, mushrooms are very filling, delicious, and super low in calories, making them a great addition to your weight loss efforts.

Carrots

Beta-carotene is a carotenoid antioxidant that gives orange fruits and vegetables their color and has powerful anti-cancer and anti-aging properties.

Carrots are excellent sources of beta-carotene, which is converted to vitamin A in the body and is essential for healthy skin, eye health, and shiny hair.

Sweet Potatoes

As with carrots, this tasty vegetable is chock-full of beta-carotene, which helps restore and regenerate damaged collagen, a major contributor to the elasticity and regeneration of our skin cells, keeping them young and supple.

Beans and Lentils

Beans and lentils are packed with protein-based amino acids to combat age related muscle loss.

Furthermore, these foods are no fat sources of protein, and so they are supportive of heart health and healthy cholesterol.

Pomegranate Seeds

Pomegranate seeds contain ellagic acid and punicalagin, both of which fight damage caused by free radicals in the body. These compounds also help preserve collagen in the skin that helps maintain a youthful appearance.

Wheat Germ

Wheat germ contains zinc, a key mineral for the production of new skin cells. Wheat germ also offers anti-inflammatory properties and may help reduce acne breakouts and prevent eczema.

A half a cup of wheat germ daily is all you need. It can be sprinkled over steamed vegetables, salads, or added to juicing, yogurt, or smoothies.

Saffron

This potent reddish spice contains two major carotenoid phytonutrients, crocin, and crocetin, two major antioxidants that have anti-tumor effects.

Saffron is believed to protect from oxidative stress and free radical damage to cells in the body. It also inhibits cancer growth factor signaling pathways, which may help stop cancer cell proliferation.

Anit Aging Drinks

Just as food is important for aging gracefully, what we drink also plays a major role in the health of our cells and organs. Here are some of the best beverages to drink on a regular basis for optimal health and vitality.

Water

We tend to forget to drink enough water, especially in the colder months. Then we start complaining of headaches, digestive problems, not being able to focus, fatigue and exhaustion. These symptoms may simply mean that you are dehydrated.

Make sure you bring a large bottle of water with you wherever you go, it may be tedious at first, but when you get used to it, you'll be glad you have it with you, as you will feel the difference.

Lemon and Lime Juice

Drinking the juice of one or two lemons or limes per day is enough to get your daily nutritional value of vitamin C. This essential vitamin is crucial for immune system and DNA health as well as younger skin with fewer wrinkles.

Cranberry Juice

Cranberries contain flavonoids that help prevent inflammation. Cranberry juice is known for treating urinary tract infections, preventing tooth decay, and improving blood circulation.

Coffee

Drinking one cup of caffeinated coffee on a daily basis may lower the risk of skin cancer. It also helps protect against type-2 diabetes, heart rhythm problems, and dementia. In addition, it boosts your energy level and helps keep you focused and alert.

Cocoa

Those who drink generous proportions of cocoa enjoy a healthier functioning of blood vessels thanks to the flavanols found in cocoa and healthy blood vessels lower risk of high blood pressure, type 2 diabetes, kidney disease, and dementia.

In a surprising turn of events, it's been proven that there is in fact, no connection between chocolate and skin problems. On an even brighter note, some types of cocoa may be considered as food for your skin.

Cocoa contains a type of flavonoid called epicatechin (so do tea and red wine). Epicatechin is vital for keeping your skin healthy since it increases blood flow to the skin, along with a good dose of oxygen supply and nutrients.

Choose quality 100% pure cocoa, not instant cocoa products.

Beet Juice

The nitrates naturally found in beets are essential for boosting blood flow to the brain, thus reducing the risk of dementia, Alzheimer's, and other diseases.

Nitrates help keep blood vessels strong and resilient, which increases the flow of blood throughout the body. Other vegetables that contain natural nitrates are **cabbage** and **radishes**.

Soymilk

Soymilk contains isoflavones, which help sustain collagen in the skin and prevent the breakdown of collagen, which is a natural part of the aging process, thus preventing the skin from sagging and losing its youthful texture.

Milk

Starting as early as in our thirties, we start to lose up to 1% of our lean muscle mass on a yearly basis. Since the amino acids found in proteins are what essentially make up our muscles, especially one known as leucine, we need to focus on getting enough of it to maintain our muscle mass, and milk does just that.

Since milk contains whey protein, which is one of the best-known sources of amino acids out there, it's crucial that we get a lot of it. Other foods that contain leucine are Greek yogurt, lean meat, soy, whey protein powder, and fish.

Your best choice in milk is grass-fed or organic viruses the conventional options because when the milk comes from cows that graze on grass instead of being fed grains by farmers, their milk will have more omega-3s and conjugated linoleic acid (CLA), which promotes bone mass, reduces body fat, and promotes immune system health.

Orange Juice

It's a well-known fact that orange juice is brimming with vitamin C, which is an antioxidant that protects the body against numerous diseases and inflammations.

Vitamin C also helps keep your skin looking vibrant and fresh. Always juice your own or choose 100% pure fresh squeezed and not sugary juice drinks.

Limit your intake, as juice is high in calories, and drink it in the morning so you can take the day to burn off those calories.

Green Tea

Green tea is great for maintaining healthy cells and protecting them against damage and stress. Packed with flavonoids, green tea helps protect against disease and block DNA damage associated with other toxic chemicals that cause destruction in the body.

It also contains theanine, which is an amino acid that helps keep you calm, focused, and less stressed. Several studies have found that pure green tea also promotes weight loss.

Always choose 100% pure green tea and not bottled green tea drinks that may contain sugar and preservatives.

Wine

Many studies have been carried out on the health benefits of moderate amounts of red wine since it contains resveratrol, a compound that may help slow down the aging process and prevent heart disease.

Also, alcohol intake in general and in moderation may protect against diabetes, memory loss linked to aging and heart disease.

Please note that the American Heart Association does not advise anyone to start drinking for heart benefits.

Here are a few tips on maintaining a good, healthy and balanced diet as you age. While it's a fact that we can't stop our bodies from aging, there are ways to slow down the aging process so you enjoy every moment of your life no matter your age.

Caloric Intake

As we age, our metabolism slows down, so we need to reduce the amount of calories we take in in order to avoid age related weight gain.

Reduce Unhealthy Fat Intake

We must reduce the amount of unhealthy, saturated fats in our diet by opting for low-fat milk and yogurt, lean poultry, fish and legumes instead of red meat that is ladled with fat.

On the other hand, eating moderate amounts of monounsaturated fats are good for you, so include these in your diet.

Some of the best sources of monounsaturated fat include

- Olive oil, peanut oil, sesame oil, canola oil, cashews, pistachios, almonds, walnuts, avocados, olives, sunflower seeds, and pumpkin seeds

Polyunsaturated fats (Omega-3 fatty acids) are also very healthy fats the body needs to thrive

- Oily fish, including mackerel, tuna or salmon, nuts and seeds such as walnuts and flaxseeds

Boost The Calcium

The risk for osteoporosis increases as the years pile on. Therefore, once we hit 50, we need to increase our calcium intake to 1200 mg daily and assess vitamin D intake.

This can help lower the risk of osteoporosis, as well as low bone mass and the overall deterioration of the bone structure.

Eating low-fat yogurt and drinking calcium-fortified orange juice are two of the best ways to get your calcium intake naturally, vitamin D supplements may also be needed, ask your doctor.

Eat Clean

Reduce or better yet eliminate processed and junk food from your diet. Eat clean, whole food created by nature and you will enjoy much better health. Refined sugar is poison to the body, so it is beneficial to also limit it or rid yourself of it altogether.

How Much Iron Do You Need?

When women are in their childbearing years, they need 18 mg of iron daily. When women reach menopause, that amount drops to less than half, only 8 mg daily, which is the same amount men need.

If you're taking a multivitamin that has iron in it, check to make sure it doesn't exceed the recommended dosage. In addition, eat foods that are naturally rich in iron, such as lean meats, beans, beef liver, and leafy greens.

Thoughts

We've probably heard it too many times to count that eating fruits and vegetables, whole grains, dairy, healthy proteins and fats, while reducing fats, sugar and salt, is key to enjoying a healthy lifestyle and preventing many types of diseases and inflammations.

However, as the years go by, we tend to forget that our bodies are well-oiled machines that need care and love to run smoothly and to stay running longer.

Just as you pay close attention to your car, smartphone, kitchen gadgets, and other tools, you need to pay close attention to your body.

The most important things are to frequently drink water throughout the day, eat the right types of food, and exercise on a regular basis.

The body changes as we age, from the way we look to how our insides work. So make sure your body maintains its zing and vitality by eating and drinking right. Your future self will thank you for it.

Foods To Eat

☐ Olive Oil & Olives

- ➢ Polyunsaturated fats

- ➢ Monounsaturated fats

- ➢ Antioxidants (vitamin E and coenzyme Q10)

- ✓ Heart Health

- ✓ Healthy Cholesterol

- ✓ Fight Damage From Free Radicals

Other Anti-Aging Oils

- Coconut Oil

- Palm Oil

- Avocado Oil

- Rice Bran Oil

☐ **Whole Grains**

> ➤ Fiber

> ➤ Beta glucans

- ✓ Heart Health
- ✓ Healthy Cholesterol
- ✓ Energy

☐ **Vitamin D Fortified Greek Yogurt**

- ✓ Bone health

- ☐ **Oysters**

  - ➢ Zinc

  - ✓ Protein synthesis

  - ✓ Immunity Health

  - ✓ Collagen Formation

  - ✓ Anti-inflammation

- ☐ **Turmeric**

  - ➢ Curcumin

  - ✓ Prevent cellular aging and degenerative diseases

  - ✓ Anti-inflammatory

  - ✓ Joint health

- ☐ **Omega-3 Fatty Acids**

  - ✓ Brain Health

  - ✓ Healthy Cholesterol and Heart Health

  - ✓ Skin Health

  - ✓ Reduction in elevated blood triglyceride levels

✓   Alleviate joint pain and stiffness from rheumatoid arthritis

✓   May help protect against dementia conditions, such as Alzheimer's disease

✓   May help prevent age related gradual memory loss linked to aging

- Walnuts

- Flaxseed and flaxseed oil

- Canola oil

- Soybean oil

- Mackerel

- Wild Caught Salmon

- Anchovies

- Bluefish

- Herring

- Sardines

- Sturgeon

- Lake trout

- Tuna

- ☐ **Dark Chocolate**

  - ➢ Flavonoids

  - ✓ Diseases prevention
  - ✓ Prevent damage from free radicals

- ☐ **Nuts**

  - ➢ Healthy fats and omega-3s

  - ✓ Immunity health
  - ✓ Prevent oxidative stress
  - ✓ Prevent cell damage
  - ✓ Prevent inflammation that accelerates aging

Perfect Portions (Choose one daily)

- 18 medium cashews
- 12 hazelnuts or filberts
- 8 medium Brazil nuts
- 12 macadamia nuts
- 35 peanuts

- 15 pecan halves

- 14 English walnut halves

☐ **Seeds**

  - ➢ Plant proteins

  - ➢ Healthy fats

  - ➢ Key nutrients for disease prevention

  - ✓ Anti-inflammation

  - ✓ Skin health

  - ✓ Heart health

  - Pumpkin Seeds

  - Sunflower Seeds

  - Flax Seeds

  - Sesame Seeds

☐ **Blueberries**

  - ➢ Key antioxidants

- ✓ Reduce risks of cancer
- ✓ <u>Reduce cholesterol levels</u>
- ✓ Reduce risks of heart disease and stroke
- ✓ May reduce risks of neurological diseases
- ✓ Brain and memory health
- ✓ Support immune system health
- ✓ Improve urinary tract health
- ✓ Improve eye health
- ✓ Prevent inflammation and oxidative damage
- ✓ Protect from free radicals
- ✓ Youthful complexion and skin health
- ✓ Positive mood

☐ **Fresh Raw Garlic**

- ➢ Key Antioxidant – Allicin

- ✓ Protection from free radicals
- ✓ Heart health
- ✓ Prevent plaque build-up in the heart
- ✓ Healthy cholesterol

☐ Kale

> Lutein

> Zeaxanthin

> Vitamin K1

> Vitamin C

> Beta carotene

> Manganese

> Copper

> B Vitamins

> Fiber

> Calcium

> Potassium

> Vitamin E

> Iron

> Magnesium

> Omega-3 fats

> Phosphorus

> Folate

✓ Prevents oxidative stress that accelerates aging

✓ Protects from damage caused by free radicals

✓ Immune system health

✓ Healthy blood pressure

✓ Healthy blood clotting

✓ Reduced risk for cancer

✓ Skin health

✓ Healthy cholesterol for heart health

✓ Contains lutein and zeaxanthin, which numerous studies have shown to greatly reduce risks for age related macular degeneration and cataracts, two of the most common eye disorders in older people

☐ Spinach

- ➤ Folate
- ➤ Beta-carotene
- ➤ Vitamin C
- ➤ Vitamin K1
- ➤ Dulforaphane

- ✓ Short-term memory health

- ✓ Reduced risk for heart disease

- ✓ Reduced risk for cancer

- ✓ Protection from free radicals

- ✓ Skin and hair health and moisture

- ☐ **Collard Greens/Salad Greens/Spinach**

  - ➢ Vitamin K1

  - ✓ Vein health and prevention of varicose veins
  - ✓ Strong bones
  - ✓ Healthy blood sugar levels
  - ✓ Healthy blood clotting
  - ✓ Prevention of heart disease
  - ✓ Possible reduced risk of Alzheimer's disease
  - ✓ Prevention of certain cancers, such as lung and liver cancer

- ☐ **Broccoli**

  - ➢ Isothiocyanates
  - ➢ Sulforaphane
  - ➢ Fiber
  - ➢ Folate
  - ➢ Vitamin K
  - ➢ Vitamin C

✓ May reduce risks for breast cancer (folate)

✓ May reduce risks for lung and colon cancer (sulforaphane)

✓ Protect from heart disease, type 2 diabetes, stroke, and hypertension (fiber)

✓ Strong bones

✓ Weight Loss

✓ Collagen production for younger looking skin (vitamin C)

Similar Foods

- Brussel sprouts
- Cauliflower
- Cabbage
- Arugula
- Watercress
- Horseradish

☐ **Swiss Chard**

> Chlorophyll
>
> Vitamin K
>
> Vitamin A
>
> Potassium
>
> Magnesium
>
> Alpha-lipoic acid

- ✓ Bone health
- ✓ Eye health
- ✓ Reduced risk for cancer
- ✓ Healthy blood sugar
- ✓ Lower blood pressure

☐ **Tomatoes**

> Lycopene

- ✓ Skin health
- ✓ Skin hydration
- ✓ Anti-wrinkle

- ✓ Protection from harmful effects of ultraviolet rays

- ✓ Heart health

- ✓ Strong bones

- ✓ Anti-cancer

- ✓ Stroke prevention

Other foods that contain lycopene:

- • Pink grapefruit

- • Carrots

- • Watermelon

- • Guava

- • Red peppers

☐ Cucumbers

- ➢ 99% water

- ➢ Silica

- ✓ Hydration for anti-aging skin health

- ✓ Anti-wrinkle and collage production

- ☐ **Soy Foods**

  - ➢ Phytoestrogens

  - ➢ Isoflavones

  - ✓ Skin health and anti-aging properties

  - ✓ Bone health

  - ✓ Heart health

  - ✓ Mimic estrogen for menopause support

    - Tofu

    - Edamame

    - Soymilk

- ☐ **Guava/Lemons/Limes/Bell Peppers/Oranges**

  - ➢ Vitamin C

  - ✓ Boost collagen production for younger skin

  - ✓ Heart health

  - ✓ Immune system health

  - ✓ Anti-Cancer

- ☐ **Black Currants**

  - ➢ Anthocyanosises

  - ✓ Eye health

- ☐ **Pineapples**

  - ➢ Manganese

  - ✓ Anti-aging skin benefits

- ☐ **Concord Grapes**

  - ➢ Polyphenols

  - ✓ Brain Health

  - ✓ Heart Health

  - ✓ Antioxidant and anti-inflammatory properties

- ☐ **Mushrooms**

  - ➢ B Vitamins

  - ➢ Vitamin D

  - ➢ Beta Glucans

- ✓ Weight management
- ✓ Reduce and prevent inflammation
- ✓ Support calcium absorption
- ✓ Anti-cancer
- ✓ Boost immunity
- ✓ Natural Detox
- ✓ Heart Health
- ✓ Healthy Metabolism

☐ **Carrots and Sweet Potatoes**

➢ Vitamin A

- ✓ Eye health
- ✓ Collagen production for younger skin
- ✓ Shiny hair
- ✓ Skin health
- ✓ Anti-cancer properties

☐ **Beans and Lentils**

> ➢ Fiber
>
> ➢ Phytochemicals
>
> ➢ Protein-based amino acids
>
> ➢ No fat protein sources

- ✓ Hair health
- ✓ Heart health
- ✓ Muscle health
- ✓ Healthy cholesterol

☐ **Wheat Germ**

> ➢ Zinc

- ✓ Skin cell production
- ✓ Anti-inflammatory properties
- ✓ Skin health
- ✓ Acne prevention

☐ **Saffron**

> ➢ Carotenoid phytonutrients: crocin and crocetin

✓ Antioxidants to fight free radicals

✓ Anti-tumor effects

✓ Prevent premature aging of DNA

✓ May help stop cancer cell proliferation

What To Drink

☐ **Water**

> ➤ Hydration that supports all internal functions within the body

☐ **Green Tea**

> ➤ Flavonoids

> ➤ Theanine

- ✓ Cell health
- ✓ Protection from free radical damage and stress
- ✓ Weight loss
- ✓ DNA health and damage protection
- ✓ Calm
- ✓ Focus
- ✓ Stress management

☐ **Lemon and Lime Juice**

> ➤ Vitamin C

✓ Boost collagen production for younger skin

✓ Heart health

✓ Immune System Health

✓ Anti-Cancer

☐ **Coffee**

> ➤ Caffeine

> ➤ Antioxidants

✓ Lower risk for cancer

✓ Focus

✓ Alertness

✓ Energy

✓ Protection from type 2 diabetes

✓ Protection from heart rhythm problems

✓ Prevent tooth decay and cavities

✓ Improved Mood

✓ Liver Health

✓ May Prevent Skin Cancer

✓ Heart Health

✓ Tightens DNA integrity

✓ Fight free radicals

☐ **Cocoa**

➢ Flavanols

➢ Epicatechin

✓ Healthy functioning of blood vessels

✓ Lower risk of high blood pressure, type 2 diabetes, kidney disease and dementia

✓ Epicatechin supports skin health, increases blood flow, oxygen and nutrients to the skin

☐ **Cranberry Juice**

> ➤ Flavonoids

✓ Anti-inflammation

✓ Tooth decay

✓ Improved

☐ **Beet Juice**

> ➤ Nitrates

✓ Boost blood flow to the brain to reduce risk of dementia diseases, and Alzheimer's disease

✓ Heart health

✓ Keep blood vessels strong

Other sources of nitrates

- Cabbage

- Radishes

☐ **Green Juice**

> ➢ Antioxidants

> ➢ Phytochemicals

> ➢ Minerals and vitamins

✓ Protection from free radical damage

✓ Protection from oxidation

✓ Healthy cholesterol

✓ Cancer prevention

☐ **Pomegranate Seed Juice**

> ➢ Antioxidants

> ➢ Ellagic Acid

> ➢ Punicalagin

- ✓ Prevent inflammation
- ✓ Reduce risks for heart disease
- ✓ Cancer prevention
- ✓ Fight damage from free radicals
- ✓ Collagen production for younger skin

☐ **Soymilk**

> ➢ Isoflavones

- ✓ Skin health and anti-aging properties
- ✓ Bone health
- ✓ Heart health
- ✓ Mimic estrogen for menopause support

☐ Milk

> Leucine

> Vitamin D

> Essential amino acids

> Calcium

✓ Bone strength

✓ Healthy muscle mass

• Leucine is also found in Greek yogurt, lean meat, soy, and fish

☐ 100% Pure Fresh Orange Juice

> Vitamin C

✓ Boost collagen production for younger skin

✓ Heart health

✓ Immune system health

✓ Anti-cancer

☐ **Red Wine or Purple Grapes**

> ➤ Resveratrol

- ✓ Slows the aging process
- ✓ Heart health
- ✓ Reduces risk for age related memory loss

☐ **Herbal Teas**

> ➤ Various compounds in support of good health

> ➤ Antioxidants

- ✓ High blood pressure
- ✓ Anti-inflammatory properties
- ✓ Stress reduction
- ✓ Prevent tooth decay
- ✓ Immune system health
- ✓ Cardiovascular health
- ✓ Blood circulation

Good Tea Choices

- Nettle tea

- Ginger tea

- Peppermint tea

- Hibiscus flower tea (sorrel)

- Green tea

- Cardamom tea

- Rosehip tea

- Blackberry leaf tea

- Hawthorn herb tea

Stay well and take care!

Tom Yeomans

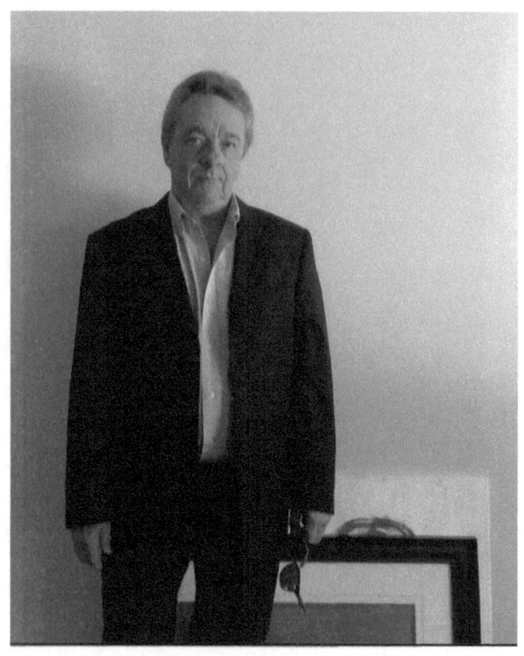

www.ingramcontent.com/pod-product-compliance
Lightning Source LLC
Chambersburg PA
CBHW031231250726
48655CB00005B/1901